THE MANE ATTRACTION

EM Moore

authorHOUSE®

AuthorHouse™
1663 Liberty Drive
Bloomington, IN 47403
www.authorhouse.com
Phone: 1 (800) 839-8640

Published by AuthorHouse 03/01/2016

ISBN: 978-1-4969-6677-3 (sc)
ISBN: 978-1-4969-6685-8 (e)

Essie Moore, M.Ed
Master Cosmetologist/Instructor

CONTENTS

ACKNOWLEDGMENT

I would like to thank everyone and the use of other relevant resources for the support during the development of this book. My husband Regenold Moore for believing in me and being there through it all, my daughter's Brittany Nichole and Tamara Marie for not giving up on their mom,and your understanding of what I have tried to accomplish has made all my efforts worthwhile. Thanks to all my friends and family for motivating and inspiring me to continue on this journey, and a special "Thank You" to Mrs. Joan Mathis, for all her help and support which has been greatly appreciated and unmeasurable. Last, but not least, I thank my Heavenly Father (GOD), who is the head of my life. Without him on my side, completing this book would not have been possible. He has given me the strength, the will, and power to go on even when I did not think I could.

"May God Bless and Keep You"
Essie

ABOUT THE AUTHOR

Hello my name is Essie Moore, a licensed Professional Cosmetologist and Instructor. I have been in the cosmetology industry for twenty plus years, and I am committed to helping others find solutions to their hair care problems. In 1986, after completing my training in cosmetology, I continued my education by receiving an Associate of Applied Science Degree in Cosmetology from Paris Junior College. I earned my Bachelors of Applied Arts & Science Degree from Southeastern Oklahoma State University and completed my Master's Degree in Education, with an emphasis on "Leadership of Educational Organizations" in 2008. I later enrolled in a program required for completing an Educational Doctorates Degree.

I am a member of the National Institute of Cosmetology. My hope is to complete my doctoral degree by the end of the year 2016, and be accepted into the "Theta Nu Sigma National Sorority."

It has been my desire to offer professional advice to those seeking a better understanding of how to provide proper care of their hair while maintaining a relationship with all cultures. It has been my experience that when it comes to analyzing the structure of the hair, I have found that "hair is hair," and it all has to be taken care of "regardless". I hope to be of help to everyone seeking advice while you are on your journey back to freedom from your hair care problems or just transitioning over from chemicals to your natural mane.

This book was written to answer professionally any questions you may have about your hair. Many people are in need of professional advice about proper hair care, how to correct problems from chemicals or just wanting to go back to their natural roots, ethnicity does not matter. This book is written to help everyone in need of answers to their haircare problems. It has been my experience, that wherever I am people are always stopping me to ask for advice on how to correct damage to their hair or how to retrieve their natural hair. Because of these instances, I was inspired to write this book as a means to reach out to others.

My Philosophy,

"Be the best,that you can be,".... and
"If you believe it, you can achieve it."

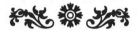

INTRODUCTION

THE MANE ATTRACTION

By Essie M. Moore

Have you ever wondered what your natural hair looks like? Guess what, I have too, so I was inspired to write this book. Many people need answers to their hair care problems, and I know that I can be of help to them, but you must first read my book. Written to help you have a better understanding of your mane, why it has changed over a period of months or years, and what you can do to retrieve its natural state.

In addition to helping you understand your mane and why it has changed, you will gain more knowledge on how to properly care for your hair when you are faced with a hair disaster from physical and chemical abuse. You will also find useful information on manicuring and artificial nails and how to properly care for them as a bonus in this book.

Instances in my life, have required me to literally stop while shopping, answer a professional question about a hair problem. The timing of the question was bad because I was in the process of taking care of my personal needs, for example, because people recognize that

I am a professional cosmetologist, they always ask questions of me, so I always try to have an answer for them.

On the other hand, I must say that it is sometimes overwhelming because they catch me off guard, and I am not really prepared to offer professional advice. This book is divided into chapters which makes it easy to read, and includes chapter-to-chapter advice on probably some of the same situations you experience on a daily basis. These suggestions are relevant for the hair care journey of any nationality.

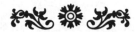

CHAPTER ONE

YOUR NATURAL MANE

"Mane is characterized as the long hair along the sides of
the neck of certain mammals, such as a horse, however; it is
also defined as a long thick growth on a human's head".

"Natural hair" refers to virgin hair whose texture remains unaltered
by the use of chemicals, hair colors, flat irons, permanent waving, and
straightening. First of all, natural hair, considered virgin hair, of birth,
whether hair cut off later in life, grows back naturally without the use
of chemicals. The texture of this natural or virgin hair for African
American people has a coarse or even softer texture than someone else's
hair even though it is all natural hair.

Hair texture defines the diameter of one single strand of hair and
is classified as coarse, medium, or fine. Hair density differs not only on
each individual, but on every strand of hair on the head. Hair texture
is best determined by simply sliding your fingers up and down the hair
strand. Your simple step will help you determine the correct texture of
your hair.

The three types of natural hair has the following characteristics:

- Coarse hair has a very resistant outer layer, and does not absorb liquids very well, require's more processing time if it were to receive a chemical service. Relaxers and permanent wave solutions are very hard to penetrate into this type of hair.
- Medium hair, considered as normal, is the easiest type to style and does not pose any problems for chemical services.
- Fine hair, the most fragile of the three (3) types is likely to abstain damage if it is not cared for properly. A way to remember fine hair is that it processes very fast and will become damaged very quickly from processing of chemicals.

The hair is made up of (3) Layers of hair. Let's take a look.

The **cuticle,** is the outside layer of the hair, has a tough outer layer which encompasses the inner layers of the hair and protects it from damage. A tough cuticle can sometimes cause problems in hair that you are trying to chemically change because it is hard to penetrate and difficult to perform any type of service. This barrier that the cuticle has around it protects it, which means that your hair is not easily broken, and it will not break down easily to receive chemical processing. Hair that has a tough cuticle is strong hair. Under a microscope the cuticle resembles fish scales. As long as the cuticle remains intact and not damaged, the hair remains protected. Exposure to the environments of the weather can change the cuticle. Exposure such as sun, water, chlorine in a swimming pool will affect the cuticle in the same way as a chemical would react on the hair that had a high alkalinity content. To perform a quick test on your hair, Take your fingers and slide them up and down the strand, if; there is no roughness about the strand, then more than likely the cuticle is intact because it does not have the feeling of roughness and it has a shiny and healthy appearance.

Located below the cuticle, the **cortex**, the second layer of the hair strand. This layer is held together by polypeptide chains connected to end bonds for strength and structure in the hair. Found just under the cuticle, is the cortex, the largest of the three layers making up approximately sixty-five to seventy percent or more of the hair, and is made up of tiny fibers which can also be affected by chemicals.

The hair is composed of Keratin, a protein made up of substances called amino acids, these amino acids form the peptide links which gives the hair strength. These links are held together by cross-bonds which are composed of amino acids, cysteine, hydrogen, and salt. In hair that is naturally straight, the peptide links are held parallel to each other by the cross bonds.

NOTICE: The hydrogen and salt bonds can be easily broken by water, (for example), when the hair has been shampooed and conditioned it can be easily damaged, due to the wringing, pulling and twisting of the hair. The hydrogen and salt bonds are the weaker bonds and lose their shape when the hair becomes wet and reshapes when the hair is dry. The salt bonds are easily broken when chemicals are applied to the hair, causing hair loss , hair dryness with loss of moisture and hair breakage.

When chemicals are applied to the hair the cross-bonds began to soften the hair and as the hair is wrapped around the perm rod, it begins to take on the shape of the perm rod. This is how the hair gets the curl definition that the clients likes, by using the size rod that is pleasing to the client. The client and the stylist together will choose which perm rod will be best suited for the clients hair and getting the curl pattern desired by both the client and the stylist. When it has completely finished processing, a neutralizer is applied to rodded hair for approximately five to ten minutes or until it locks and re-hardens the curl into its new position. This procedure has permanently changed your hair into a curly or wavy position.This process is usually found amongst caucasian or asian nationalities. However; ethnic people can obtain similar results.

In chemical hair relaxing, it is just the opposite, the relaxer is applied and the hair is combed straight; the cysteine links are softened, allowing the peptide links to become parallel. The neutralizer or fixative is applied, and the cysteine links reharden, holding the hair straight permanently.This method is usually performed on ethnic or African American hair.

A little about haircoloring…it is also a chemical process. The pigment found in the cortex, is called melanin, which is made up of black, yellow, red, or brown melanin pigments or color. These pigments are affected by any haircolors that you choose to use on the hair, and when the hair begins to turn gray, that is a sign that the melanocytes have stopped producing melanin. Hair normally turns gray as a sign of the natural aging process and it can also occur at any age, or may be present at birth. Heredity normally plays the main factor which determines when a person's hair will begin to turn gray, although illness, shock, and stress can also play a major factor.

The *medulla*, innermost layer of the hair, is sometimes absent and poses a problem for some hairstyling products to be effective, this includes haircutting, hairstyling, and chemical services, especially those used in permanent waving.

Did you know?

Did you know that the hair is composed mainly of a protein called keratin, which is located in all horny growths including the nails and skin and the chemical composition of hair varies with its color. The hair is divided into two different parts, the root and the shaft. The hair root is that portion of hair located beneath the skin, this portion of the hair extends above the skin. The papilla is located at the bottom of the hair follicle and fits into the hair bulb. Inside the hair papilla are blood and nerve supply that contribute to the growth of the hair. As long as you have a healthy papilla the hair will grow normal and allow new hair to grow. Diet also influences the general health of the hair. Eating too many sweets, starches, and fatty foods can cause the sebaceous glands to become overactive and secrete too much sebum.

Maintaining your Natural Hair:

Now that your natural hair structure has been explained, let's take a look at how to maintain your natural look. In order to maintain your natural hair structure, you must not chemically change your hair. If chemicals are used on the hair, it becomes chemically altered.
Think Back: Remember the three layers of hair, the cuticle, cortex, and medulla. Applying chemicals, however, alters permanently the structure of the hair.

Proper care of your natural hair' would be to shampoo and condition at least twice a week, to rid the hair and scalp of any hairspray and build-up of oils. Make sure that you massage the scalp area when shampooing to stimulate the blood vessels, which promote good hair growth.

Myth: Oily scalp promotes hair growth, and "is" there such a thing as "Growing Dandruff"?

Absolutely False: Oily scalp is caused from a buildup of oil and sebum on your scalp and slows down the growth process because the hair follicle gets clogged, and the hair cannot grow properly. It either grows in thin patches or not at all which will soon result in becoming bald in those untreated areas of the head.

African Americans usually have a growth pattern of curly hair, and the hair that grows out of the hair follicle is usually oval or flat, although some suggest that definite reasons exist why the hair grows naturally curly. Some even suggest that ethnic hair grows faster on one side, than the other side, because of the way that you sleep. It is suggested that the side that you sleep on the most will grow the slowest and become shorter than the other side, however; there is no evidence that supports this theory. My professional guess would be that, "If" the hair is growing slower on the "sleepy side", and breaking off, it is because the hair is losing it's moisture from the bedding soaking it up and causing stress to that side of the head from the position that the body is laying. This could possibly cause damage to your hair at some point and time.

Let's discover what causes dandruff. Don't forget about the myth! Dandruff, is caused by excess shedding and dying of the skin cells on the scalp begins when flaking takes place. As the new skin cells are renewed on the scalp the old dead skin cells are pushed out and replaced. Dandruff can be controlled by using a gentle shampoo, and if the dandruff is severe enough use a medicated shampoo for dandruff control. Dandruff does not promote hair growth; it actually hinders the growth of the hair because it needs proper care by simply cleansing the hair to allow the hair and scalp to breathe properly.

To maintain that natural curl pattern, African American Women use good moisture balanced products because the hair loves water and moisture which helps to prevent the hair from becoming dry and brittle.

After shampooing and conditioning towel dry the hair and apply a moisture balanced product to the hair. After towel drying, leave enough water in the hair after towel drying the hair to absorb the moisture product. You will need to experiment with how much product you will need to apply to the hair in order to have good results. Let the hair naturally dry and re-apply if needed until you have enough moisture in the hair and you can see the curl in the hair. Trim your hair about once a month to get rid of split ends

Remember: Your hair is naturally curly and it should have a natural curl or wave pattern if you follow these instructions. After shampooing and conditioning the hair it will appear dry and nappy looking, but after following this procedure, the hair begin to curl up. For effective results, repeat this procedure after each shampoo.

For Caucasian and Asian hair, the procedure to maintain your beautiful mane is to shampoo and condition the hair, using a leave in conditioner mainly because of blow drying the hair, this helps to prevent split-ends and hair breakage. When blow-drying the hair use a product that has little alcohol content, and apply as little tension as possible, helping to prevent shedding, and damaging the hair. Trim the hair about once a month to promote proper hair growth and use a light holding spray, if needed for hold.

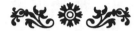

CHAPTER TWO

BRAIDS AND HOW TO PROPERLY CARE FOR THEM

Let's Take a Look:

Many styles can be created by Hair braiding, braiding is an art that originated centuries ago and has been used by many and it is even more popular today. Some say that hair braiding originated in Africa and others claim that it originated in Egypt and it is now one of the fastest growing trends in the beauty industry today. The cost of braiding is very expensive and range in price from $100.00 to $250.00 dollars a head depending on the geographical area in which you live. It also depends on the type of braids that you have requested, it usually requires a sitting time of about 8-to-12 hours. Not to mention that once the hair has been completed, some styles require an additional 1½-to-2 hours to perhaps trim the ends, seal the ends, and style the hair. Using synthetic hair usually has the longest lasting style because synthetic hair does not slip or open up on the ends of the natural hair when it is shampooed.

Braids should not be worn for a period of no longer than 8 weeks because it stresses the hair when it is twisted for a long period of time. Some of the types of braids are box braids, micro braids, cornrows, senegalese and tree braids. There are many types of braids however; the care of braids would basically be the same.

Follow this plan to properly care for your mane:

Follow the hair care advice received from your stylist and be sure to ask questions. Be sure you fully understand how to care for braids of any type while you have them, and whenever you decide it is time to remove them.

Shampoo your hair and scalp regularly with a professional shampoo (ask your stylist to recommend a shampoo) for your hair type, and condition the hair while it is braided.

Some stylists recommend waiting a month before the first shampoo and conditioning treatment, the individual decides how often he/ she would like to shampoo the hair. After thoroughly shampooing, conditioning and rinsing the hair, apply a leave-in conditioner to the hair, and a braiding spray is recommended to help the hair retain moisture. Damage will occur to the edges of the hair if not cared for properly. A scalp oil must be applied around the edges to prevent damage. There are a number of products available to assist the customer with hair problems, such as using pure store bought olive oil around the sides of the hair, tea tree oil, and vitamin- e. Constant contact with the stylist will allow your hair can be monitored as you wear this easy going and long lasting style.

Care of the Braids
- Do not allow braids to remain too tight in the hair especially around the edges. If too tight ask stylist to loosen the braid. Too much tension will eventually destroy your hair follicle.
- Notice any bumps around the edges, which may suggest that the hair is stressed and too tight. Remove the braids immediately.

- Do not allow braids to remain in the hair more than eight weeks or two months to avoid any complications and damage to your hair.
- Remove the braids gently, preferably by a professional. Remember the hair is in a fragile state and will break easily.
- Shampoo the hair and massage to loosen and thoroughly cleanse the hair and scalp. Follow with a protein treatment to help strengthen and replace moisture.

Myth: Braiding makes the hair grow longer and fuller.

Absolutely False: Braiding does not allow your hair to grow longer and fuller. Braiding like any other hair style that requires maintenance, has a lasting effect on the hair and allows the client to maintain that style for a period of time. After the braids are removed a great amount of shedding will occur.

Tension will cause permanent hair damage to your hair follicles. The edges are the most sensitive to braiding because the braids are pulling against the scalp. Pulling the hair up into different styles such as wearing pony tails and pinning the hair up causes stress to the edges of the hair and the center part of the head. Notice that whenever you wear braids the top center of your head becomes very sore and you may not understand the reasons for the soreness. Most of the time, a stylist gets caught up in making the client look good, and when she is in that frame of mind, the scalp and the edges of the hair suffer.

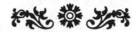

CHAPTER THREE

CHEMICALLY TREATED HAIR

News You Can Use

Chemical Hair Relaxing is the process of *permanently* rearranging the basic structure of over-curly hair into a *straight* position. Chemical Hair Relaxing should be administered under the supervision of a licensed professional. Products are available to the public, however the manufacturer "still" recommend that the products be administered by a licensed professional.

Of the two types of hair relaxers, sodium hydroxide and ammonium Thioglycolate. Sodium hydroxide is the most commonly used in salons today. Sodium hydroxide, a caustic relaxer ranges on a PH scale from 10 to 14. "Lye" is the common household name. The sodium hydroxide relaxer has both a swelling and softening action on the hair. As the relaxer penetrates the hair and absorbed the bonds in the hair are broken. By using the comb, or the hands to smooth the hair begins to straighten. To prevent hair breakage do not apply to much tension or pressure when manipulating the product onto the hair. When applying this particular product, work with speed and be cautious of the time spent in applying the product. The allotted amount of time to leave sodium hydroxide in the hair is approximately 8 to 10 minutes, depending on the hair texture; fine hair may require less time. If the product is left too long on the hair, the hair will become brittle and dry. The hair at this stage is damaged and must be treated or cut off where damaged. Reconditioning treatments are recommended after any relaxer has been applied to the hair.

On the other hand, Ammonium Thioglycolate is a type relaxer that is less drastic for the hair and is used to relax over-curly hair. This chemical is used when a client wishes to have even a more manageable curl. Ammonium Thioglycolate is used to soften and then the hair is wrapped around perm rods to re- shape the natural curl pattern in the hair. A neutralizer is used to harden the curl to its new shape; the hair is then rinsed and moisturizer applied. This style usually lasts approximately 3 -to -4 months.

It is not recommended for hair, that has been recently tinted, lightened, hot combed, or treated with a metallic dye should not be chemically changed with sodium hydroxide or ammonium Thioglycolate; to do so would damage or destroy your hair completely. The only option would be to cut the hair off and start over. This precaution should be followed when applying ammonium:

- Do not apply this chemical (ammonium thio), to hair that has been relaxed with sodium hydroxide. The hair will not curl because the hair has been *permanently* rearranged with sodium hydroxide into a straight position.

A person with virgin hair or natural hair (hair that has no chemicals on it) should use caution when using chemicals on your hair. For example: your hair is natural, but your hair is too tight and curly, and you want to soften it or make your hair more manageable. You go to the beauty supply and purchase a product that states that you can use this product on men and women to loosen the *natural locks, but the* product that you just purchased contains *calcium hydroxide* or *sodium hydroxide,* All right, "You just put a relaxer back into your hair," because you did not understand the ingredients. You are no longer natural and have put a chemical back into your hair that you have worked so hard to remove. Understanding manufactured ingredients is of utmost importance when you are applying chemicals to your hair. You should always seek professional guidance to perform any chemical service.

Can you remember when you got your first Relaxer/perm on your hair?" You're probably like me" and you just don't remember. It was probably when your mother thought your hair was too hard "nappy" to comb anymore and she put a relaxer in your hair when you were probably four or five years old. So, you really don't know what your real natural hair looks like, do you? Because you can't remember at such a young age, is why so many people are desiring to find an answer for their hair care problems and get back to the mane attraction. They want to understand what to do with their natural mane, but do not have an idea of what their natural/virgin hair ever looked like. Using chemicals on the hair is the answer for some people, but for those that have a greater desire to know what their natural hair really looks like, applying chemicals is not the answer.

Perform this quick test on yourself to help you determine what your natural hair is supposed to look like. Do not apply a chemical to your hair for 12- or more weeks. You will begin to see about ½ to 2 inches of curly or wavy hair, called new growth. This hair is your new mane growing out of your hair follicle in its natural state and this is what your natural mane would look like without chemicals

A Word of Caution:

- Always examine the scalp and hair for abrasions before applying chemicals.
- Put on protective gloves to protect the hands.
- Understand the product and always follow the manufacturer's directions.
- Use caution to avoid getting chemicals into the eyes, on the skin, and in the ears.
- Do not apply a Thio relaxer over a sodium hydroxide relaxer and vice –versa.
- Shampoo and condition the hair thoroughly after removal of product.
- Do not pull or twist your hair when applying the relaxer.
- Apply a protective base to prevent scalp and chemical burns.
- Shampoo the hair at least three times when removing relaxer from the hair.
- Always use a neutralizing shampoo when removing a relaxer from the hair.

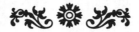

CHAPTER FOUR

HAIR COLORING

Let's take a look:

Hair coloring, the art of changing your natural hair color which involves adding artificial color to the pigments in the natural hair, thus changing the hair color. Hair lightening on the other hand involves the complete removal of pigment from the hair.

Let's take a look:

- A Hair coloring rinse is a certified hair color and is applied after you have completed the shampoo. It is applied directly after shampooing and left in the hair. It is combed through and blow-dried or roller set in the hair. When the hair is shampooed the next week, the rinse washes out in the shampoo. Must be put back into the hair after each shampoo to maintain color.

- Highlighting shampoos enhances your hair color, eliminating the dullness and brightening any color on your hair.

- Hair color crayons comes in the form of sticks like a crayola in all different shades. They are made from synthetic waxes and soaps, and are normally used in between hair coloring treatments to keep the gray from showing through. This type of color is messy and dulls easily, losing it's potency.

- Hair color sprays come in a spray can and in various shades, and are sprayed directly onto the hair to cover up gray or add tones to the hair. This type of color comes out on your hands, scalp, and anything that it comes in contact with.

- Mascara is not a hair color for your head, but for the face and is used on the eyelashes to enhance a person's appearance making their eyelashes appear fuller and longer.

- Semi-Permanent Tints are formulated to last from four to six weeks. These colors do not require the use of a developer. They are self-penetrating and are applied without developer. Because they primarily set on the surface of the cuticle, they do not open the cuticle of the hair, but mainly coat the hair shaft causing a color change.

- Notice: Semi-colors will not lift your hair at all. They will darken but they will not lift your hair color to a lighter shade.

- Permanent hair color usually last six to eight weeks and penetrates deep into the hair. It permanently changes your hair color. Different developers are used with this hair color. Most of the time, if the color is purchased at a local store you will find that the permanent color contains two bottles in the box which is the tint and the developer. In most hair color boxes, you will find 20- volume developer. Manufacturers hardly ever put anything stronger than 20 -volume in a box of hair color. However, when you purchase a more professional hair color at your beauty supply, thorough knowledge must be taken to make sure that you purchase the correct color and choose the correct developer. The professional hair color normally stands alone in a beauty supply store, so you have to remember that you must choose a developer to go with the hair color. In a beauty supply, you have 20, 30, 40, and even 50 volume developer. If you are not a professional stylist, you should seek the advice of a professional before purchasing ad applying any hair color.

- Metallic Dyes contain lead acetate and silver nitrate and are never used professionally. They coat the hair shaft and render it unsatisfactory for any type of service leaving the hair brittle and hard. The hair appears to have a greenish cast left from the silver nitrate and a purple cast left from the lead in the hair. In order to remove metallic dyes, you should seek professional advice and follow manufacturer's directions.

A Word of Caution:

Perform a patch test in order to make sure that you are not allergic to product. This test can be performed by placing a very small amount of hair color on a cotton ball or tip and slightly rubbing the color onto the skin behind the ear. Do not disturb the area for 24 hours before washing off with shampoo and thoroughly rinsing the area until clean, if no reaction continue with your service. However, if any signs of swelling, inflammation or redness occurs, those are signs of allergic reaction and by no means should you continue with the service.

When you test for color selection a strand test must be performed, note that this is different from a patch test. To perform the strand test you should check to determine whether the hair is strong enough to do the service and has porous areas. To perform the test mix a small amount of tint with 20 volume developer. Apply the tint to a strand of hair, allow it to remain on the hair until shade is reached. After shade is reached, wash and dry the strand and examine the hair. If you are satisfied with results observing no signs of breakage, you can proceed with the service.

- Always wear protective gloves.

- Do not apply color to the hair if signs of abrasions are present on the scalp.
- Do not brush your hair prior to hair coloring service.
- Always read manufacturer's directions before applying hair color.
- Always perform a strand test before coloring the hair.
- Always perform a patch test before coloring the hair.
- Do not use metal containers or implements when performing hair color service.
- Use a mild shampoo, to prevent stripping off the hair color.
- Protect your clothing form hair color stains.
- Seek the advice of a professional before performing any hair color.

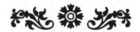

CHAPTER FIVE

THERMAL HAIR STRAIGHTENING

"From the Oldie Way of Straightening to the Newbie"

Thermal Hair straightening, commonly known as Hair Pressing used to be a service in demand. However, over the years hair pressing has diminished and the flat irons have evolved for all types of hair. Thermal hair pressing requires the use of a stove, pressing comb, and pressing oil. Before performing this service, a scalp and hair analysis should be administered. There are two types of pressing combs involved in hair pressing, the electric iron and the regular stove top irons. Preparing the hair for thermal pressing and using the flat iron is the same procedure and if caution is not taken, when performing either service, you will suffer hair damage.

Thermal Pressing Procedure: Must not be performed on Chemically Relaxed hair
Let's take a Look:

For Ethnic hair only
Do not thermal press Caucasian or Asian hair using a heating stove and pressing comb, but you may use flat irons (optional).

- Make sure to turn the irons on before the service, and set the temperature if possible.
- If using the stove top irons, turn stove on prior to the service and lay out your straightening comb on a clean dry cloth.
- Divide the hair into small one-quarter sub-sections.
- Test the temperature of the irons on a white sheet of paper.
- Apply a small amount of pressing oil to the hair.
- Lift the hair and begin to insert the pressing comb into the hair
- Run the comb through from scalp to hair ends.
- Repeat until all sections are complete.

Flat Irons Procedure: Can Be Performed on Chemically Relaxed Hair

Although there are no chemicals involved in flat ironing, there are still risk involved when using heat on the hair.

Let's take a closer look:

Caucasian and Asian hair may follow this method
- Before using flat irons always begin with clean hair.
- Adjust the flat irons to correct temperature.
- Check temperature of irons on a white sheet of paper or cloth. (If cloth turns brown, readjust the irons before inserting them into the hair).
- You do not want any type of hairsprays or spritz in the hair.
- You may spray a heat protectant on the hair as you are using the irons and you may apply a hair silken product, such as; silk therapy to help smooth the end and make the hair softer.
- A heat protectant protects the hair from any damage.
- Remove any tangles from the hair to ensure a smooth finish to the hair.
- Pull the irons through the hair from scalp to hair ends.

- Repeat this process until your hair is silky straight.
- Clean your irons with thermal iron cleaner and wipe off thoroughly.
- Do not use Oil sheen and Hair sprays and spray directly onto your flat irons, these products could possibly damage your mane, start a fire, be caustic, and hazardous to your health.

Notice: Flat irons getting hotter than others, does not mean that they are the best. As a matter of fact, they are the worst because they get too hot and "fry" your hair.

What to do when your hair has been damaged from using excessive heat:
- Shampoo the hair with a moisturizing conditioning shampoo.
- Condition with a deep penetrating conditioner.
- Section and trim off the split, burnt, or brittle ends.
- Continue this procedure at least once a week until hair is healthier and shows signs of improvement.

Remember hair-is-hair and it does not take *frying* heat to smooth your hair cuticle. Using a flat iron with a heat control device will allow you more freedom to apply heat as needed. Try this method for better results.

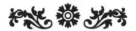

CHAPTER SIX

HAIR EXTENSIONS

Hair extensions make an individual's hair look more appealing or more stylish. However, have you ever wondered why after wearing the extensions for a period of time you begin to lose your hair or maybe your hair begins to thin in certain areas.

Let's take a look.

Hair extension is a method used to temporarily make the hair look fuller, longer, and more attractive. However, hair extensions can cause a great deal of hair damage. They come in human hair and synthetic. The human hair extensions are usually the most expensive and the synthetic cost the least amount of money. Synthetic hair extensions are pretty, but you cannot iron curl or flat iron this type of hair. It is made of chemical fibers and already has some shape to it before you use it. Hair extensions come in various colors and vary in length.

- When deciding which type of hair would be best for you, first examine the condition of the hair and scalp.
- When selecting your extensions, you must decide on the style that you are wanting to achieve and then choose the correct package of hair for that particular service. Keep in mind that all types of adornment, if not cared for properly, will damage

your hair, whether by bonding, which is using a bottle of hair bonding glue and spreading the bond onto the weft and attaching it to the root of the hair. Another method of applying hair extensions is called hair fusion, this method is done by using heat to the tip of the extension and fusing onto the hair.

- Hair clippers/combs is also a quick do it yourself, at home method. The hair extensions come pre-made to use. Remove the extensions from the package and adjust the comb to insert into the hair, clamp it, and you are ready to go.
- The hair tape extensions is also a method of applying extensions to the hair. This method requires the proper tape strips in order to make this a successful outcome. The tape is pressed onto the weft and the natural hair, finger press across the strand to ensure proper fit.
- The sew-in method, another method requires braiding the hair into corn rows or some type of braid, and the extension is then sewn on the braid with a needle and thread.

Regardless of the method chosen, you should seek professional advice when applying hair extensions because you could suffer temporary to permanent hair loss.

"Let me explain."

Hair is an appendage of the body's skin. It is a slender thread-like outgrowth of the body. No nerves are present in the make- up of the hair there; the hair has no sense of feeling. The main purpose of hair is for protection from heat, cold, injury, and facial features. In order for the hair to stay healthy and beautiful, you must take good care of it. Abusing the hair by using chemicals, braiding and hair extensions should all be considered. The hair is made primarily of a protein called keratin, also present in other body parts, such as, the nails.

The hair follicle encases the root of the hair and is a tube like depression in the scalp. Every strand of hair on the human head has a hair follicle, and one or more oil glands are attached to each follicle. The mouth of the hair follicle is the breeding place for germs and the accumulation of sebum, sweat, and dirt. When bonding glue, tape adhesive, and dirt get into the follicle and clogs it, the hair cannot grow properly, thus causing thinness in whatever area this problem exists, meaning if the hair is left untreated, temporary hair loss will become permanent loss of hair. When the hair is healthy the hair grows and has a radiant shine, but if the body is ill, the hair weakens. When the bloodstream provides the hair papilla with food elements, the hair grows properly.

What Causes Permanent Hair Loss

Let's take a closer look:

Permanent hair loss is usually caused by the genetic makeup of the human body, called male- pattern baldness and female- pattern baldness. You have inherited your parent's genes, and whatever the genes are at the time of conception is what your hair will be like. It is almost like you have no control over it. You cannot change your genetic makeup, so you have to live with whatever you have been handed down from generation to generation. It's that simple. You can't change it, so you have to learn to adapt and do whatever you have to do to make it work for you.

Genetic hair loss is a direct result of your hormones. There are products on the market today, that will help with this problem, but if your parents are genetically bald and lost their natural hair at a young age then more than likely, you will too. Testosterone is the most important factor in a male's hair growth. Testosterone is a male sex hormone that is important for sexual and reproductive development. Women also produce this hormone but at a lower level. When the testosterone accumulates in the blood vessels leading to the growth of the hair. It overpowers the hair follicle and kills it. The only thing that you can do is look into getting a hair transplant if you are a male, and for women use products that are available for baldness. Such as, Rogaine, it has a medicine in it for hair called monoxididil and is the only medication on the market at this time to promote hair growth. Losing the hair is from the shrinkage of the hair follicle, and when that happens you get thin, fine, and less hair growth which will eventually result in permanent hair loss.

Other factors that contribute to hair loss:

An accumulation of oils and sebum on the scalp, dirt, pollution, and styling products suffocates and kills the hair follicle. It is probably clogged with all of the above and the result is the loss of your hair. One of the main things that causes of baldness in men is the wearing of a cap of some sort or a covering over the scalp. This causes the scalp to sweat, build up oils and dirt, again destroying your hair follicle. Individuals that wear Pony tails or hair attachments in the top of their head usually complain of hair baldness or bald patches because the hair is stressed and pulled in a direction that it does not want to be pulled. The hair wants to just hang down and be free to relax and move as it should and the way it grows. Men normally trying to ward off cowlicks and their receding line with different products by brushing and combing, usually aggravates the problem, and causing even more baldness.

Malnutrition is another cause for hair loss. The hair needs vitamin supplements, protein, minerals, and good nutrition to grow properly, stay strong and healthy. Scalp massaging may be an answer to some of our hair problems, although it has not been proven. When you perform scalp massages, it causes the scalp to turn from white to pink which indicates that the blood vessels are being stimulated which may in turn bring some nutrients to the hair follicle and help promote hair growth. Tip: Scalp massaging can't hurt so you might give it a try and check out the results.

Other factors that contribute to hair loss are chemicals, medication, radiation, chemotherapy, diseases and stress. There are (2) factors listed above that could be reversed with proper care of the hair and body.

- Stress can be brought on by many factors, employment, medical reasons, emotional problems or anything that may worry you.
- Drugs like methamphetamines will cause you to lose your hair temporarily. There are other drugs that will cause hair loss such as, drugs that are used to treat cancer, depression, high blood pressure, heart disease, depression and arthiritis.

- Diet plays a big part in healthy hair growth, and so do nutrients and vitamins, along with proper shampooing and conditioning.
- Thyroid problems regulates hormones, and if gland is not working properly will cause hair loss.
- Skin condition called "Lupus" or Lichen Planus causes scarring on the scalp, resulting in permanent hair loss where the scars are present.

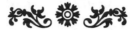

CHAPTER SEVEN

NAILS

Did you know that when you are having any service performed on the nails, careful consideration must be taken due to nail diseases and infections that could occur.

Let's take a look:

Performing a manicure requires the professional knowledge of a nail technician or a licensed cosmetologist. The first step in getting a manicure is that you want to first, make sure that all of your implements are clean, have been sanitized and disinfected. This will prevent the spread of infection while performing the service. The next step in a manicure is to always examine your hands for any abrasions or irritation that may be present. If no abrasions or irritation is present, you will proceed with your manicure. If you are using your tools repeatedly make sure that your tools have been disinfected thoroughly. Be careful when storing your implements because this can set up a breeding ground for bacteria-even it's your own stuff. There is a method that is approved for all salons in the state of Texas that can help you in deciding the product's that you can use to completely disinfectant your implements.

According to the Texas Department Rules and Regulations, rule 83: Health and Safety Standards-Department-Approved Disinfectants. (a)

EPA –registered bacterial, fungicidal, and virucidal disinfectants shall be used as follows: Implements and surfaces shall first be thoroughly cleaned of all visible debris prior to disinfection. EPA registered bactericidal fungicidal, and virucidal disinfectants become inactivated and ineffective when visibly contaminated with debris, hair, dirt, and particulates…..and…(b)-1. Chlorine bleach at the appropriate concentration is an effective disinfectant for all purposes in a salon.

When performing a manicure use these quick and easy steps:

Always begin the service with clean hands and disinfected implements.
- Remove the old polish from the nails by soaking your nails with a cotton ball that has been soaked in non-acetone nail polish remover and remove the old polish.
- File your nails from corner to center, this prevents the sawing motion of moving back and forth. This sawing motion tears away the nails and makes them split at the free edge and disrupts the nail plate which will cause splitting and peeling.
- Caution: Never file nails that have been soaking in water because this makes the nails to soft and this also causes the nails to be easily broken and split when filing.

Do not file into the corner of the nail because this can cause an infection to occur.

When the skin is removed or pulled away from the nail, it allows room for bacteria to grow. Just start at the corner and file to the center. Without pushing into the corners of the skin.
- Immerse the nails into warm soapy water.
- Apply cuticle softener to each nail and push back the cuticle with a cuticle pusher or an orange wood stick. Nippers may be used to nip the nails, this helps to remove dead skin from

around the cuticle. (Nippers must be used with caution-follow manufacturer's direction).

- Put your hands back into the soapy water and brush across your nails. This removes the dead cuticle form pushing and nipping the nails.
- Rinse the nails and dry them.
- Apply lotion and perform hand and arm massage.
- Clean under the free edge with a cotton tipped orange wood stick.
- Remove lotion from the nail plate with a cotton ball with non-acetone polish.
- Apply basecoat and then apply top coat at least to coats of polish.
- Clean and disinfect your area and implements for use again.

Pedicures are performed in similar manner as a manicure, except for product usage.

Notice signs of ingrown nails on the feet and be aware if you are a diabetic, due to cutting around your cuticles with nippers. Could possibly cause injury, if so, (seek the advice of a physician immediately). All injuries should be treated by a physician.

Artificial nails

Artificial Nails are very popular. They can make your hands look very attractive and they are long lasting. Nail tips require fills about once every two -to -three weeks. They range in cost from twenty dollars for a full set, to approximately 60 dollars a full set. It depends on the type of service you are requesting. When you go to a professional about getting a new set of artificial you should make sure that you wash your hands before the service. This helps cut down on the spread of germs and bacteria. The technician should always have disinfected implements before beginning the service. The implements that are being used on you should not be used on another client. For instance: Bacteria from the previous person is present on the nail file, and if it is used on another individual, it spreads the bacteria., which can cause serious illness, such as, mold on the nails, fungus, loss of a nail or the entire finger, and may be required to use antibiotics for a period of time. There have been confirmed and reported instances where clients have visited salons and had to seek medical attention from a professional because they got infected from the use of unsanitary implements. Due to these instances State laws were rewritten regulating better sanitary practices in the beauty industry. She was treated for infections for about a year. The Texas Department of Licensing and Regulations in 2006 amended their health and safety standards on manicuring and pedicuring services, to include that cosmetologist and manicurists shall wash their hands with soap and water or a hand sanitizer prior to performing any services, and that all implements must be cleaned, sanitized, and disinfected prior to a client's service. If a buffer block or porous nail file is exposed to broken skin or unhealthy skin or nails, it must be discarded immediately after use in a trash receptacle.

Today's concerns revolve around resistant bacteria called staphylococcus aureus. It is a type of staph infection that is resistant to antibiotics and very hard to get rid of. Bacteria is always on the body, but you and your own body are in tune with each other. If your bacteria is transferred to another person through an open sore or cut it could cause serious illness for that person.

A word of caution on pedicures: Do not get a pedicure if you have open wound, scratches, or skin irritation microorganism's lives in footbaths and can enter through any break in the skin.

When using different products on the nails and feet, such as, nail polishes, base and top coats, hand lotions etc., it should all be used in a professional manner. When giving or receiving a nail polish service, polish that has been used on the feet should never be used on the hands, although this is what most people do, it is unsanitary because the nail polish brush has been used on the feet.

Remember: Nail polish has a number of solvents in it which makes it really tough and resistant to house germs and bacteria, therefore; growth is not possible.

I hope that this book has helped you to understand some of the way's to help assist on your journey to becoming natural and wearing your "MANE" proudly. I also, hope that the bonus addition of this book has offered you some insight on proper care of the nails.

NOTICE TO THE READER

This book is designed to help offer an understanding of your hair textures, whether it is Ethnic hair, Asian hair, Caucasian hair or whatever type hair there may be. It only offers suggestions and tips to the reader. It is not to solve any of your hair care problems. It does not guarantee any of the products described herein or perform any independent analysis connection with any of the product information contained herein. The publisher of this book does not assume responsibility or obligation for any services that you choose to use from this book. The book is solely to be used as an informational guide to help you understand more about your hair and your nails.

The publisher or the author shall not be liable for any special, consequential, or exemplary damages resulting, in whole or part, from the readers' use of, or reliance upon, book. The author and the publisher assumes no responsibility for anything that you might read or try in this book.

HAIR TYPE CHART

Classifications: 1-4

Class 1	Class 2	Class 3	Class 4
Straight hair	Wavy	Curly	Kinky
"No other pattern than straight"	2a-Slightly wavier	3a-Slightly curly	4a-Very curly
	2b-More Wavy	3b-More curly	4b-Curlier, zigzazzy appearance.
	2c-Waviest	3c-Even more Curly	4c-Very tight curl pattern, no curl pattern hardly visible.
Notes:			

COSMETOLOGY TERMS FOR YOUR MANE

African American- Black or African American.

Asian- A native or inhabitant of Asia.

Axillary-Refers to hair that grows under the arm.

Barba- Refers to hair on the face.

Bleach-Product that strips the layers of the hair. It usually turns from brassy orange-red to high yellow and white.

Capilli-Refers to hair on the scalp.

Caucasian-of or relating to the white race of humankind as classified according to physical features

Cilia- Refers to the eyelashes.

Cortex-Middle layer of the hair, located directly beneath the cuticle layer. The cortex is responsible for the incredible strength and elasticity of the hair.

Cuticle-The outermost layer of hair, consisting of a single, overlapping layer of transparent, scale-like cells.

Haircolor- artificial color that changes your natural haircolor

Hair Density-Refers to how close your hair grows on your head.

Hair-texture-Hair can be defined a coarse, medium, or fine. The cuticle determines the texture of the hair.

Lanugo or Vellus Hair-Refers to body hair, sometimes called "baby" hair.

Mane-long, thick hair growing from the neck of a horse or around the neck of a lion. b.) Long, thick hair on a person's head

Medulla-Innermost layer of the hair, composed of round cells, often absent in the hair

Melanin-Tiny grains of pigment deposited in the basal layer of the epidermis and papillary layers of the dermis.

Nationality-the status of belonging to a particular nation, whether by birth or naturalization.

Pubic-Refers to genital hair.

Supercilia-Refers to the eyebrows of the face.

Printed in the United States
By Bookmasters